SAVORING

WELLNESS

COOK BOOK

20 DIABETIC GOURMET RECIPES AFTER 50

FOR BEGINNERS

MOH LIMS

Copyright©2023 Moh Lims

All right reserved

Table Of Content

INTRODUCTION

One constant in the colorful fabric of life is our love for food. We congregate around tables, experiencing the pleasures of food and the warmth of shared moments.

But what if, in the middle of our gastronomic experiences, we could also make decisions that benefit our health, particularly as we approach our golden years?

Thank you for visiting "Savoring Wellness: The Diabetic Gourmet - Recipes After 50." This cookbook is a symphony of delectable possibilities, constructed with age-old knowledge and taste mastery. It's a book that will captivate your senses, stimulate your taste buds, and equip you with the knowledge you need to make mindful, health-conscious decisions.

Consider relishing a delectable Grilled Lemon Herb Chicken that is properly seasoned and tender while also knowing that it will help you on your diabetes control path. Consider a beautiful Asian-Inspired Salmon Bowl, a brilliant celebration of nutrition and flavor, while you take responsibility of your health in style.

Consider the joy of sharing a hearty bowl of Lentil and Vegetable Soup as you embrace a lifestyle that feeds both the body and the spirit.

Our cookbook is a culinary journey for adults over the age of 50, a celebration of life's richness and the knowledge that comes with age. Inside, you'll find a treasure trove of recipes that have been meticulously handpicked to satisfy the special dietary demands of diabetics, all while offering an explosion of tastes and textures that will make your taste buds dance with ecstasy.

But "Savoring Wellness" is more than simply a cookbook. It's a compass pointing you in the direction of a better, more vibrant existence. We'll start on a voyage of discovery with each meal, learning about the advantages of mindful eating and the delights of feeding our bodies and spirits.

So, whether you're an experienced home cook or a culinary newbie, come along with us on this wonderful journey. We'll discover the secrets of bright, tasty, and health-conscious cooking together. It's time to appreciate wellness, mature gracefully, and leave a culinary legacy that honors both the love of food and the love of life.

Let's go on this tasty adventure together, since the pleasure of eating properly knows no age, and the skill of experiencing wellness begins with the first mouthful.

1: Grilled Lemon Herb Chicken

Ingredients:

- 4 boneless, skinless chicken breasts
- 2 lemons, juiced and zested
- 2 cloves garlic, minced
- 2 tablespoons fresh rosemary, chopped
- 2 tablespoons fresh thyme, chopped
- Salt and pepper to taste

Instructions:

- ❖ Combine lemon juice, lemon zest, minced garlic, rosemary, thyme, salt, and pepper in a mixing bowl.

- ❖ Pour the marinade over the chicken breasts in a resealable plastic bag. Refrigerate for at least 30 minutes after sealing the bag.

- ❖ Heat the grill to medium-high.

- ❖ move the chicken from the marinade and grill for 6-8 minutes each side, or until the internal temperature of the chicken reaches 165°F (74°C).

❖ Serve immediately with steamed broccoli or a mixed green salad.

Benefits:

❖ Because this recipe is minimal in carbs, it is excellent for diabetics.

❖ Lemon adds a blast of flavor without adding extra sugar.

❖ Fresh herbs give antioxidants and taste richness.

2: Roasted Vegetable Quinoa Salad

Ingredients:

- 1 cup quinoa, rinsed and drained
- 2 cups mixed vegetables (bell peppers, zucchini, cherry tomatoes)
- 2 tablespoons olive oil
- 1 teaspoon dried oregano
- Salt and pepper to taste
- 1/4 cup feta cheese (optional)
- 1/4 cup balsamic vinaigrette dressing

Instructions*:*

- ❖ Preheat the oven to 400 degrees Fahrenheit (200 degrees Celsius).

- ❖ Toss together the mixed veggies with the olive oil, dried oregano, salt, and pepper. Distribute them on a baking pan.

- ❖ Roast the veggies in the oven for 20-25 minutes, or until soft and slightly browned.

- ❖ Meanwhile, cook the quinoa according to the package directions.

- ❖ Combine the cooked quinoa and roasted veggies in a large mixing dish.

- ❖ Drizzle with balsamic vinaigrette and sprinkle with feta cheese (optional).

- ❖ Serve hot or cold.

Benefits*:*

- ❖ Quinoa is a low-glycemic grain that aids with blood sugar regulation.

- ❖ Roasted veggies contain fiber and vital minerals.

❖ Balsamic vinaigrette provides taste without adding too much sugar.

3: Spicy Chickpea and Spinach Curry

Ingredients:

- 2 cans (15 oz each) chickpeas, drained and rinsed
- 1 onion, chopped
- 2 cloves garlic, minced
- 1 can (14 oz) diced tomatoes
- 2 cups fresh spinach
- 2 tablespoons curry powder
- 1 teaspoon cayenne pepper (adjust to taste)
- 1 tablespoon olive oil
- Salt and pepper to taste

Instructions:

❖ In a large pan over medium heat, heat the olive oil.

❖ Add the chopped onion and sauté for 3-4 minutes, or until transparent.

- ❖ Combine the minced garlic, curry powder, and cayenne pepper in a mixing bowl. Cook for an additional 1-2 minutes.

- ❖ Stir in the chopped tomatoes and chickpeas. Cook for 10-15 minutes.

- ❖ Add the fresh spinach and heat until it has wilted.

- ❖ Season with salt and pepper to taste.

- ❖ Serve with brown rice or cauliflower rice as a side dish.

Benefits:

- ❖ Chickpeas are high in protein and fiber, which can help keep blood sugar levels stable.

- ❖ Spinach is abundant in iron and other critical minerals.

- ❖ Spices offer taste without the use of sweets or salt.

4: Baked Salmon with Dill Sauce

Ingredients:

- 4 salmon fillets

- 1 lemon, thinly sliced

- 2 tablespoons fresh dill, chopped

- Salt and pepper to taste

Dill Sauce:

- 1/2 cup plain Greek yogurt

- 2 tablespoons fresh dill, chopped

- 1 tablespoon lemon juice

- 1 clove garlic, minced

- Salt and pepper to taste

Instructions:

- ❖ Preheat the oven to 375 degrees Fahrenheit (190 degrees Celsius).

- ❖ Season the salmon fillets with salt, pepper, and dill. Top with lemon slices.

- ❖ Wrap each fillet in aluminum foil and place in the oven for 15-20 minutes, or until the salmon flakes easily with a fork.

- ❖ While the salmon bakes, make the dill sauce by combining all of the sauce ingredients in a mixing dish.

- ❖ Top the roasted salmon with a dab of dill sauce.

Benefits:

- ❖ Salmon is high in omega-3 fatty acids, which are good for heart health.

- ❖ Greek yogurt has protein but no additional sugars.

- ❖ Dill provides taste without adding salt.

5: Berry and Almond Smoothie Bowl

Ingredients:

- 1 cup unsweetened almond milk

- 1 cup frozen mixed berries

- 1/2 banana

- 1 tablespoon almond butter

- 1 tablespoon chia seeds

- Fresh berries and sliced almonds for topping

Instructions:

* ❖ Blend together almond milk, frozen berries, banana, almond butter, and chia seeds in a blender.

* ❖ Blend until the mixture is smooth and creamy.

* ❖ Transfer the smoothie to a bowl.

* ❖ Garnish with fresh berries and almond slices.

* ❖ Serve immediately.

Benefits:

* ❖ This smoothie bowl is strong in fiber and low in added sugars.

* ❖ Berries include a lot of antioxidants and vitamins.

* ❖ Almonds include both healthful fats and protein.

6: Quinoa-Stuffed Bell Peppers

Ingredients:

- 4 large bell peppers, any color

- 1 cup quinoa, rinsed and drained

- 1 can (14 oz) black beans, drained and rinsed

- 1 cup diced tomatoes

- 1/2 cup corn kernels (frozen or canned, no added sugar)

- 1 teaspoon chili powder

- 1/2 teaspoon cumin

- Salt and pepper to taste

- 1/4 cup shredded low-fat cheddar cheese (optional)

Instructions:

- ❖ Preheat the oven to 375 degrees Fahrenheit (190 degrees Celsius).

- ❖ Remove the tops of the bell peppers and discard the seeds and membranes.

- ❖ Toss together quinoa, black beans, chopped tomatoes, corn, chili powder, cumin, salt, and pepper in a large mixing dish.

❖ Place each bell pepper in a baking tray and stuff with the quinoa mixture.

❖ Bake for 25-30 minutes, covered with aluminum foil.

❖ Remove the cover, sprinkle with cheese, and bake for another 5 minutes, or until the cheese is melted and bubbling.

❖ Serve immediately.

Benefits:

❖ Quinoa is a low-glycemic grain that is strong in protein and fiber.

❖ Bell peppers are abundant in vitamins and antioxidants. This meal has a lot of plant-based proteins.

7: Zucchini Noodles with Pesto

Ingredients:

- 4 medium zucchinis, spiralized into noodles

- 1 cup fresh basil leaves

- 1/4 cup pine nuts

- 2 cloves garlic, minced

- 1/4 cup grated Parmesan cheese

- 1/4 cup olive oil

- Salt and pepper to taste

- Cherry tomatoes for garnish (optional)

Instructions:

- ❖ Combine basil, pine nuts, garlic, Parmesan cheese, olive oil, salt, and pepper in a food processor. To prepare the pesto sauce, blend everything together until smooth.

- ❖ Heat a little amount of olive oil in a large pan over medium heat.

- ❖ Add the zucchini noodles and cook for 2-3 minutes, or until just soft.

❖ Take the pan off the heat and combine with the pesto sauce.

❖ If preferred, garnish with cherry tomatoes.

❖ Serve right away.

***Benefits*:**

❖ Zucchini noodles are a low-carb alternative to pasta.

❖ Basil and garlic in the pesto sauce add flavor without adding sugar.

❖ This dish is low in carbohydrates and high in healthy fats.

8: Baked Eggplant Parmesan

***Ingredients*:**

• 2 medium eggplants, cut into rounds

• 2 cups tomato sauce (no added sugar)

• 1 cup shredded part-skim mozzarella cheese

• 1/4 cup grated Parmesan cheese

• 1/4 cup chopped fresh basil leaves

• 2 tablespoons olive oil

Instructions:

* ❖ Preheat the oven to 375 degrees Fahrenheit (190 degrees Celsius).

* ❖ Drizzle olive oil over eggplant slices and season with salt and pepper.

* ❖ Arrange the eggplant slices on a baking pan and bake for 15-20 minutes, or until cooked, flipping halfway through.

* ❖ Layer tomato sauce, eggplant slices, mozzarella cheese, Parmesan cheese, and chopped basil in a baking dish, repeating until all ingredients are utilized.

* ❖ Add a layer of cheese on top to finish.

* ❖ Bake the cheese for 20-25 minutes, or until it is bubbling and brown.

* ❖ Allow for a few minutes of rest before serving.

Benefits:

* ❖ Eggplant is low in carbs and high in fiber, while tomato sauce is high in lycopene and vitamins. This meal is a diabetic-friendly take on a traditional Italian dish.

9: Lemon Garlic Shrimp and Asparagus

Ingredients:

- 1 pound big peeled and deveined shrimp

- 1 bunch asparagus, trimmed and sliced into bite-sized pieces

- 2 tablespoons olive oil

- 2 cloves garlic, minced

- zest and juice of 1 lemon

- salt and pepper to taste

Instructions:

- Toss together the shrimp, asparagus, olive oil, chopped garlic, lemon zest, lemon juice, salt, and pepper in a mixing dish. To coat, toss with a fork.

- Melt the butter in a large pan over medium-high heat.

- Cook for 4-5 minutes, or until the shrimp turn pink and opaque, in the pan with the shrimp and asparagus mixture.

- Garnish with fresh parsley, if desired.

❖ Serve immediately.

Benefits:

❖ Shrimp is a lean protein source, and asparagus is low in carbohydrates and high in nutrients.

❖ Lemon and garlic give flavor without the use of sugar.

10: Greek Salad with Grilled Chicken

Ingredients:

- 2 boneless, skinless chicken breasts
- 1 cucumber, diced
- 1 cup cherry tomatoes, halved
- 1/2 red onion, thinly sliced
- 1/2 cup pitted and sliced Kalamata olives
- 1/2 cup crumbled feta cheese
- 2 tablespoons olive oil
- 2 tablespoons red wine vinegar
- 1 teaspoon dried oregano

Instructions:

- ❖ Heat the grill to medium-high.

- ❖ Season the chicken breasts with olive oil, dried oregano, salt, and pepper to taste.

- ❖ Grill the chicken for 6-8 minutes each side, or until it reaches an internal temperature of 165°F (74°C).

- ❖ Thinly slice the cooked chicken.

- ❖ Toss together diced cucumber, cherry tomatoes, red onion, Kalamata olives, and crumbled feta cheese in a large mixing basin.

- ❖ Drizzle with olive oil and vinegar. To mix, toss everything together.

- ❖ Garnish with grilled chicken pieces.

- ❖ Serve right away.

Benefits:

- ❖ The salad is loaded with fresh veggies and healthy fats, and the Greek flavors provide flair without adding sweetness.

11: Lentil and Vegetable Soup

Ingredients:

- 1 cup washed and drained dry green or brown lentils

- 2 carrots, diced

- 2 celery stalks, chopped

- 1 onion, chopped

- 2 garlic cloves, minced

- 1 can (14 oz) chopped tomatoes (no added sugar)

- 6 cups low-sodium vegetable broth

- 1 teaspoon dry thyme

- Salt and pepper to taste.

Instructions:

- ❖ Sauté onions, carrots, and celery in olive oil in a large saucepan until tender.

- ❖ Stir in the garlic, thyme, salt, and pepper. Cook for 1 minute more.

- ❖ Pour in the lentils, diced tomatoes, and vegetable broth. Bring the water to a boil.

❖ Reduce the heat to low, cover, and cook for 30-40 minutes, or until the lentils are cooked.

❖ Garnish with fresh parsley and serve hot.

Benefits:

❖ Lentils are high in protein and fiber, which help to balance blood sugar levels.

❖ This soup is low in fat and salt.

❖ Vegetables are high in nutrients.

12: Cauliflower and Broccoli Stir-Fry

Ingredients:

• 1 small head cauliflower, chopped into florets — 2 cups broccoli florets

• 1 sliced red bell pepper

• 2 minced garlic cloves

• 2 tablespoons low-sodium soy sauce

• 1 tablespoon sesame oil

• 1 teaspoon minced ginger

• 1/4 cup chopped green onions

- optional crushed red pepper flakes

- sesame seeds for garnish

***Instructions**:*

- ❖ Heat sesame oil in a large pan or wok over medium-high heat.

- ❖ Stir in the minced garlic and ginger for 1 minute.

- ❖ Stir in the cauliflower, broccoli, and red bell pepper. Stir-fry the veggies for 5-7 minutes, or until they are tender-crisp.

- ❖ Toss in the low-sodium soy sauce to coat.

- ❖ Garnish with chopped green onions, crushed red pepper flakes, and sesame seeds, if preferred.

- ❖ Serve immediately with brown rice or cauliflower rice.

***Benefits**:*

- ❖ Cauliflower and broccoli are low-carb veggies high in vitamins and fiber, and this stir-fry is a healthier alternative to takeout.

❖ Sesame oil and ginger provide flavor without the need of additional sweeteners.

13: Turkey and Vegetable Skewers

Ingredients:

- 1 pound lean ground turkey

- 1 zucchini, split into rounds

- 1 yellow bell pepper, chopped

- 1 red onion, chopped

- 1 teaspoon dried oregano

- 1 teaspoon garlic powder

- Salt and pepper to taste

- Soaked wooden skewers

Instructions:

❖ Combine lean ground turkey, dried oregano, garlic powder, salt, and pepper in a mixing bowl.

❖ Make tiny meatballs out of the seasoned turkey mixture.

❖ Alternately thread the turkey meatballs, zucchini rounds, yellow bell pepper pieces, and red onion chunks onto the wooden skewers.

❖ Heat a grill or grill pan on medium-high.
❖ Grill the skewers for 8-10 minutes, turning every now and then, until the turkey is cooked through and the veggies are soft.

❖ Serve immediately.

Benefits:

❖ Lean ground turkey is a low-fat protein source; vegetables give fiber and important minerals; and this meal is low in carbs and good for diabetics.

14: Cucumber and Avocado Salad

Ingredients:

- 2 cucumbers, thinly sliced

- 2 ripe avocados, diced

- 1/4 red onion, thinly sliced

- 2 tablespoons fresh cilantro, minced

- 1 lime juice • 2 tablespoons olive oil

Instructions:

- ❖ Combine thinly sliced cucumbers, diced avocados, thinly sliced red onion, and chopped cilantro in a large mixing dish.

- ❖ Drizzle with olive oil and lime juice.

- ❖ Season to taste with salt and pepper.

- ❖ Gently toss to mix.

- ❖ Serve cold.

Benefits:

- ❖ Cucumbers and avocados are low in carbohydrates and high in healthful fats.

- ❖ This salad is hydrating and refreshing.

- ❖ Lime juice and cilantro enhance flavor without including any extra sweeteners.

15: Spinach and Mushroom Stuffed Chicken Breast

Ingredients:

- • 4 boneless, skinless chicken breasts

2 cups fresh spinach, chopped

- 1 cup mushrooms, finely chopped

- 2 garlic cloves, minced

- 1/4 cup low-sodium chicken broth

- 1/4 cup grated Parmesan cheese

- Salt & pepper to taste

Instructions:

- ❖ Preheat the oven to 375 degrees Fahrenheit (190 degrees Celsius).

- ❖ Sauté minced garlic and mushrooms in olive oil in a pan until the mushrooms shed their moisture and become soft.

- ❖ To the pan, add the chopped spinach and chicken broth. Cook until the spinach begins to wilt.

- ❖ Remove from the heat and add the grated Parmesan cheese. Season with salt and pepper to taste.

- ❖ Butterfly each chicken breast carefully and fill with the spinach and mushroom mixture.

- ❖ Use toothpicks or kitchen string to secure.

* ❖ Transfer the filled chicken breasts to a baking tray.

* ❖ Bake for 25-30 minutes, or until the chicken is well done.

* ❖ Before serving, remove the toothpicks or string.

Benefits:

* ❖ Spinach and mushrooms offer fiber and vitamins to this meal, which is low in carbs and heavy in protein.

* ❖ It's a tasty and filling alternative for diabetics.

16: Baked Sweet Potato Fries

Ingredients:

* 4 big peeled and chopped sweet potatoes

* 2 tablespoons olive oil

* 1 teaspoon paprika

* 1/2 teaspoon garlic powder

* Season with salt and pepper to taste

Instructions:

* ❖ Preheat the oven to 425 degrees Fahrenheit (220 degrees Celsius).

* ❖ Toss sweet potato fries with olive oil, paprika, garlic powder, salt, and pepper in a large mixing dish until equally coated.

* ❖ Arrange the fries on a baking sheet in a single layer.

* ❖ Bake for 20-25 minutes, or until the fries are crispy and golden, turning halfway through.

* ❖ Serve immediately.

Benefits:

* ❖ Sweet potatoes are a good source of fiber and vitamins.

* ❖ Baking reduces the overall fat content compared to frying.

* ❖ This side dish is lower in carbohydrates than traditional potato fries.

17: Asian-Inspired Salmon Bowl

Ingredients:

- 4 salmon fillets

- 2 cups cooked brown rice

- 1 cup steamed broccoli florets

- 1/2 cup shredded carrots

- 1/4 cup low-sodium soy sauce

- 2 tablespoons rice vinegar

- 1 tablespoon honey or a sugar alternative

- 1 teaspoon grated ginger

Instructions:

- ❖ Heat the grill to medium-high.

- ❖ Season the salmon fillets with salt and pepper to taste.

- ❖ Grill the salmon for 4-5 minutes per side, or until it is cooked through.

- ❖ Whisk together soy sauce, rice vinegar, honey (or sugar alternative), and grated ginger in a small pot. Cook over low heat until it thickens somewhat.

* Divide cooked brown rice, steamed broccoli, shredded carrots, and grilled fish among serving dishes.

* Drizzle the sauce over the bowl and top with sesame seeds, if using.

* Serve immediately.

Benefits:

* Salmon contains omega-3 fatty acids, which are beneficial to heart health.
* Brown rice is a complex carbohydrate that can help balance blood sugar. This meal is high in protein, healthy fats, and fiber.

18: Berry Chia Seed Pudding

Ingredients:

* 1 cup unsweetened almond milk

* 1/2 teaspoon vanilla extract

* 1 cup mixed berries (strawberries, blueberries, raspberries)

* 1 tablespoon slivered almonds (optional)

Instructions:

- ❖ Combine chia seeds, unsweetened almond milk, and vanilla extract in a mixing dish. Stir well.

- ❖ Refrigerate the mixture for at least 4 hours or overnight, stirring regularly, until it thickens.

- ❖ Layer the chia seed pudding with mixed berries before serving.

- ❖ If preferred, garnish with slivered almonds.

- ❖ Serve cold.

Benefits:

- ❖ Chia seeds are high in fiber and healthy fats, while berries are high in antioxidants and low in sugar.

19: Beef and Vegetable Stir-Fry

Ingredients:

- 1-pound lean beef strips (sirloin or flank)
- 2 cups broccoli florets

- 1 sliced red bell pepper

- 1 thinly sliced yellow onion

- 2 minced garlic cloves

  - 2 tablespoons low-sodium soy sauce
  - 1 tbsp sesame oil 1 tbsp cornstarch (or sugar alternative) 1/4 cup low-sodium beef broth Salt & pepper to taste

Instructions:

- ❖ Whisk together soy sauce, sesame oil, cornstarch (or sugar alternative), and beef broth in a small bowl.
- ❖ Brown the meat in a large pan or wok over high heat. Set aside after removing from the skillet.

- ❖ In the same skillet, heat a little amount of oil and stir-fry the broccoli, red bell pepper, onion, and chopped garlic until tender-crisp.

- ❖ Return the cooked meat to the pan and drizzle with the sauce.

❖ Continue to stir-fry for another 2-3 minutes, or until everything is completely coated and cooked through.

❖ Season to taste with salt and pepper.

❖ Serve immediately.

Benefits*:*

❖ Lean beef adds protein without adding fat; vegetables give vitamins and fiber; and this stir-fry is a low-carb supper choice.

20: Greek Yogurt Parfait

Ingredients*:*

• 1 cup Greek yogurt, plain

• 1/2 cup mixed berries (strawberries, blueberries, raspberries)

• 1/4 cup chopped nuts (almonds, walnuts, or pecans) — 1 tablespoon honey or sugar alternative

• 1/2 teaspoon vanilla essence

Instructions*:*

❖ Combine plain Greek yogurt and vanilla essence in a mixing dish.

- ❖ 2. In a glass or dish, layer the yogurt with mixed berries and chopped almonds.

- ❖ Drizzle honey (or a sugar alternative) on top.

- ❖ If preferred, garnish with a dusting of cinnamon.

- ❖ Serve cold.

Benefits:

- ❖ Greek yogurt has a lot of protein and probiotics, while berries include antioxidants and natural sweetness.

- ❖ Nuts give crunch and healthy fats.

CONCLUSION

As we near the end of "Savoring Wellness: The Diabetic Gourmet - Recipes After 50," we hope you've discovered not just a wonderful selection of recipes, but also a key to unlocking the door to a healthier, more vibrant existence.

This cookbook is more than simply a collection of recipes; it's a road map to wellness prepared exclusively for diabetics over the age of 50.

You've been through a world of flavors in these pages, from the spicy Grilled Lemon Herb Chicken to the warm embrace of Lentil and Vegetable Soup. With our Asian-Inspired Salmon Bowl, you've discovered the delight of thoughtful eating, as well as the refreshing simplicity of a Cucumber and Avocado Salad.

You've realized that eating healthily doesn't have to mean foregoing flavor; it means relishing both healthiness and the delights of the table.

The advantages you've learned from "Savoring Wellness" go beyond the kitchen. With this cookbook in your possession, you've gained:

Better Blood Sugar Control: Our recipes are carefully designed to assist regulate blood sugar levels, allowing you to enjoy meals without experiencing unwanted spikes.

Heart Health: Many of our recipes contain heart-healthy components such as salmon, olive oil, and whole grains, which promote cardiovascular fitness.

Weight treatment: You'll find meals that encourage a healthy weight, which is important in diabetes treatment.

Nutrient-Rich Meals: Each meal is meant to supply critical nutrients, vitamins, and minerals, therefore improving overall health.

Variety and Flavor: "Savoring Wellness" introduces you to a variety of flavors, guaranteeing that eating healthily is never boring or repetitive.

Confidence in the Kitchen: Whether you're a seasoned chef or just starting out, our simple instructions and useful hints can help you improve your cooking abilities.

A Culinary Legacy: By embracing the ideas of "Savoring Wellness," you're leaving a legacy of healthy cooking for yourself and your loved ones.

Remember that the path to wellness is a continuing one when you close this cookbook and return to your own kitchen. Every meal is an opportunity to make health-promoting decisions that may be both nutritious and genuinely pleasurable. You've equipped yourself with information, and you now have the means to produce culinary masterpieces that promote your health.

We encourage you to keep exploring the realm of mindful eating, experimenting with new foods, and relishing every meal. Thank you for including "Savoring Wellness" in your culinary adventure. May your future meals be filled with health, pleasure, and the delectable tastes that only life after 50 can provide.

You are savoring wellness with each meal, not simply eating. Good appetite!

Savoring Wellness - Because Life Is Meant to Be Enjoyed at Any Age.